Essential Oils Blends
30 Recipes To Feel Full Of Energy And Look Well-Groomed

Table of Contents

Introduction

Nature has gifted us with innumerable blessings in the form of natural resources and a lot of valuable items. The unprecedented beauty of earth has been embellished further with various resources like wind, water, minerals and other botanical sources.

The purpose of all these creations is to serve various needs of humans, in such a way that the life of human race can continue with any kind of interruption or deficiency. However, the responsibility of appropriate use for all these resources lies with us so that the eventual benefit of all these useful creations can be gathered in the best possible way.

Among the resources which can be a true treasure for us, essential oils come as most prominent treasures for our use. Extracted from a number of various botanical species, essential oils are usable for a number of various purposes including therapeutic, aromatic and remedial.

As the use of artificial and processed materials, both for food and medicine has put us in a number of side effects. It is because of this reason, that the use of natural ingredients and supplies is being focused in past few years. Essential oils have also attracted the attention of experts and researchers who have found that essential oils if explored and utilized genuinely can be the real treasures for our lives.

Chapter 1 – Essential oils - a miraculous gift of nature

If you look around in your vicinity, you can't see anything better than natural remedies. It is because nature's principles are the most suitable ones for mankind. Essential oils also come as one of those miraculous gifts of nature which are best suitable for mankind. Looking at the below-mentioned recipes you will come to know the diverse range of utility of these essential oils.

1. Citrus Blend Massage oil

Ingredients:

- Ylang Ylang essential oil- 10 drops
- Spearmint essential oil -25 drops
- Peppermint essential oil - 5 drops
- Bergamot essential oil – 10 drops

Directions:

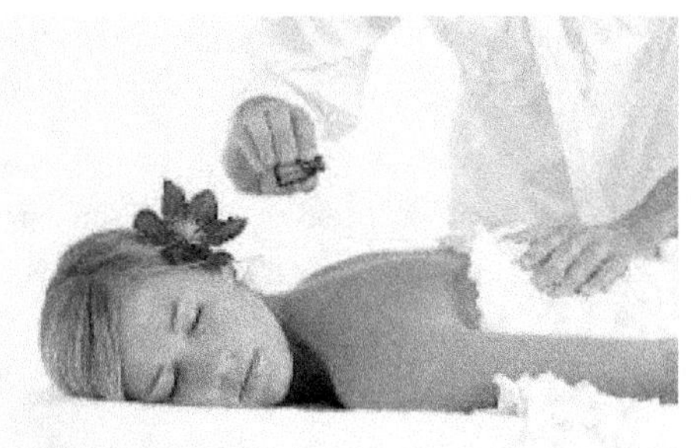

The primary utility of this recipe will be gained by the sunlight treatment, which will be accomplished by putting the oil bottle in sunlight. The essential oils mentioned in this recipe are all useful for gaining excessive energy when they come in contact with the particular composition of sunlight. It will make the oils more useful. Put together all of the mentioned essential oils in an appropriately sized bottle.

Shake the bottle in circular motions so that all of the ingredients are mixed together. Make sure that you do not fill up the bottle up to the lid. It will leave some of space for shaking the ingredients before every use. The Ylang Ylang essential oil present in the ingredients is an important ingredient for soothing your nerves and enhancing your energy. So this mixture is best suitable for massage purpose.

2. Herbal mix for blood purification

Ingredients:

- ➢ Thyme essential oil - 15 drops
- ➢ Ginger essential oil - 15 drops
- ➢ Marjoram essential oil - 20 drop
- ➢ Bergamot essential oil – 10 drops

Directions:

Take up all of the ingredients together in an appropriately sized bottle. Shake the bottle in circular motions so that all of the ingredients are mixed together. Make sure that you do not fill up the bottle up to the lid. It will leave some of space for shaking the ingredients before every use. The Oregano essential oil present in the

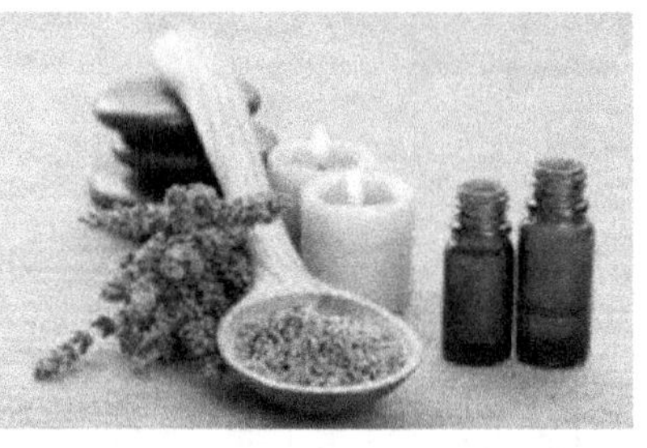

ingredients is an important ingredient for blood purification so all the problems which emerge because of blood issues can be greatly reduced if this herbal mix is used on regular basis. .

3. Basil essential oil for shower floor

Ingredients:

- ➢ Thyme essential oil - 20 drop
- ➢ Oregano essential oil - 5 drops
- ➢ Marjoram essential oil - 10drop
- ➢ Basil essential oil –5 drops

Directions:

Put together all the ingredients in an appropriately sized bottle. Shake the bottle in circular motions so that all of the ingredients are mixed together. Make sure that you do not fill up the bottle up to the lid. It will leave some of space for shaking the ingredients before every use.

The Basil essential oil present in the ingredients is an important ingredient for adding a sweet aroma which will enhance your bathing experience. After you are done with regular bath, add few drops of this mixture on your palm and rub over the skin. It can be sued for the whole body easily.

4. Bergamot essential oil for uplifting

Ingredients:

- ➢ Peppermint essential oil - 15 drops
- ➢ Bergamot essential oil - 20 drops
- ➢ Orange essential oil – 20 drops
- ➢ Lemon essential oil - 10 drops

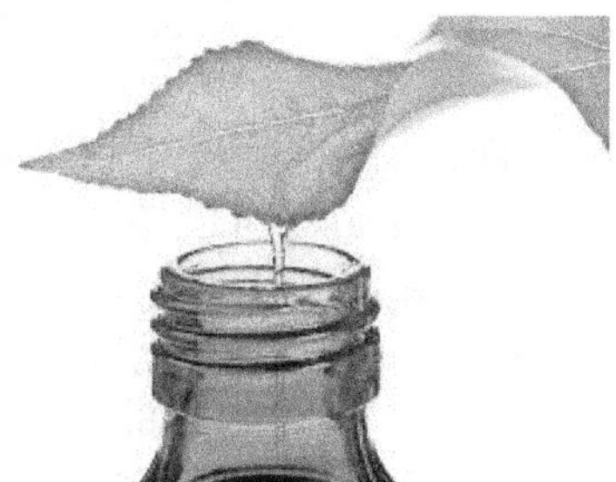

Directions:

Take a bottle of transparent color and add all the ingredients in this bottle. Thoroughly mix all the ingredients and spin off the bottle well. Place the bottle at room temperature. Placing in sunlight will allow all the extract to mix well.

Now use this mixture for people who have lower levels of energy or higher level of depression, which hinders their productivity. The best time for using this mixture is at night so that you can have a comfortable sleep and wake up energetic without any kind of irritation or anger.

5. Weight defeating Clary Sage essential oil

Ingredients:

- Marjoram essential oil - 10 drops
- Lemon essential oil – 20 drops
- Clary Sage essential oil - 15 drops

Directions:

Put together all the ingredients in an appropriately sized bottle. Shake the bottle in circular motions so that all of the ingredients are mixed together. Make sure that you do not fill up the bottle up to the lid. It will leave some of the space for shaking the ingredients before every use. The Clary Sage 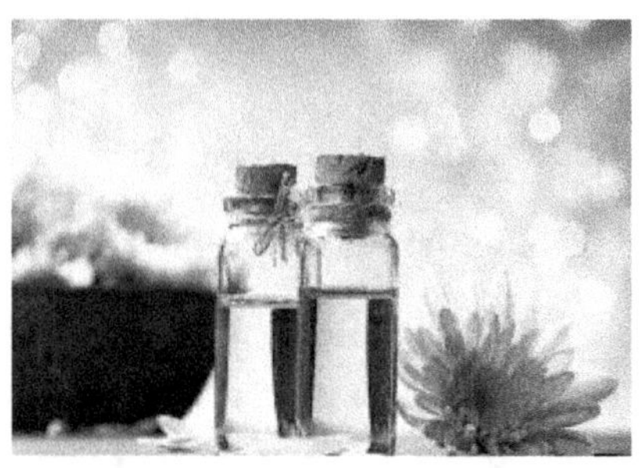 essential oil present in the ingredients is an important ingredient for lowering down of weight but do not use it in excessive quantity. It will be useful when you use it in recommended quantity.

6. Get sporty energy with Marjoram essential oil

Ingredients:

> - Peppermint oil - 12 drops
> - Marjoram essential oil- 20 drops
> - Dill seed essential oil - 15 drops
> - Bergamot essential oil – 40 drops

Directions:

The primary utility of this recipe will be gained by the sunlight treatment, which will be accomplished by putting the oil bottle in sunlight. The essential oils mentioned in this recipe are all useful for gaining excessive energy when they come in contact with the particular composition of sunlight. 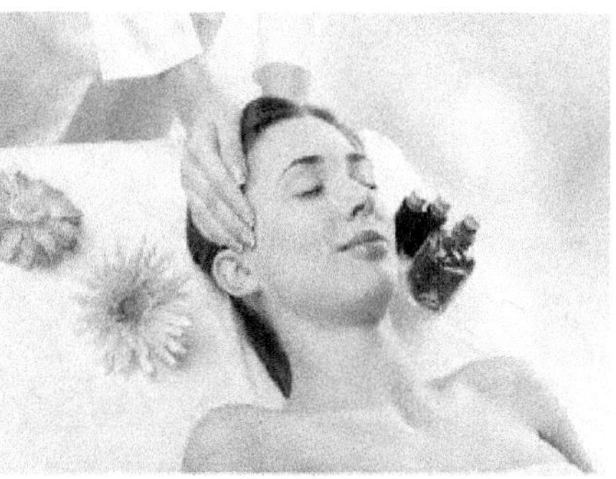 It will make the oils more useful. Put together all of the mentioned essential oils in an appropriately sized bottle. Shake the bottle in circular motions so that all of the ingredients are mixed together.

Make sure that you do not fill up the bottle up to the lid. It will leave some of the space for shaking the ingredients before every use. The Peppermint essential oil present in the ingredients is an important ingredient for gaining of energy, especially for sports activities. But excessive amount used can be troublesome, so do not add it more than the prescribed quantity.

7. Immunity gain with Fennel essential oil

Ingredients:

> ➢ Thyme leaves (minced) – 1/4 cup
> ➢ Fennel essential oil - 20 drops
> ➢ Water- 2 cups
> ➢ Ginger (crushed) – ¼ cup

Directions:

In a large pan add water. Heat the water till you can see bubbles coming out. Put crushed ginger and turn the flame to medium. Let the ginger settle down in the hot water for ten minutes. It will make all the extract of ginger 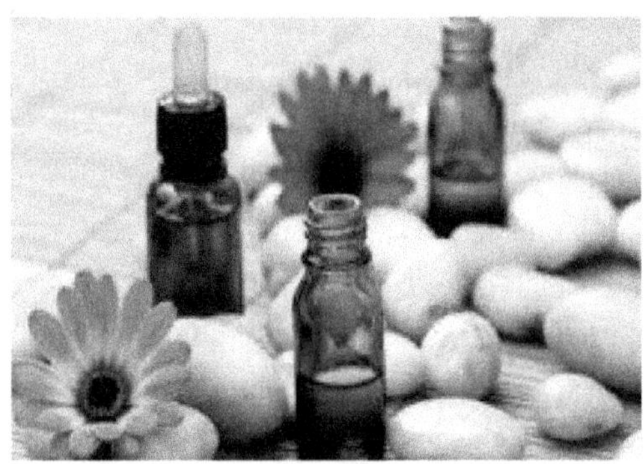 to get settled and thoroughly mixed in water. Let water get evaporated till the quarter of the original quantity. Meanwhile, prepare a glass bottle by rinsing it with hot water and salt mixture. Let it get dry.

Now pour all the mixture of ginger in the bottle and fill it up fully with Fennel essential oil. Leave bottle in sunlight. Use two drops of this extract daily. It will enhance your immunity levels and if you get successive bacterial or viral attacks, this mixture can be very much helpful for you. It will also increase the overall vitality of the body.

8. Ginger essential oil for weight loss

Ingredients:

- Thyme essential oil - 10 drops
- Ginger essential oil - 15 drops
- Water- 2 cups
- Peppermint essential oil – 5 drops
- Cinnamon powder – 2 teaspoon

Directions:

Get hold of a pan in which you can add up the mentioned quantity of water. But make sure that you do not make the flame too high. It will evaporate the water too quickly. Heat over low flame, until visible bubbles appear in boiling water. Now add cinnamon powder and let the mixture boil extensively.

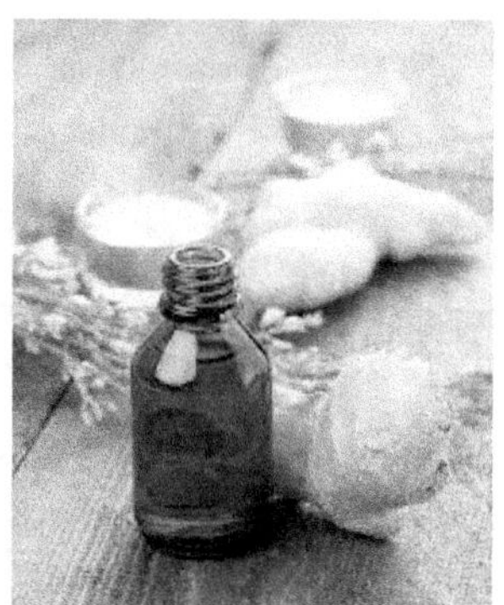

Turn the heat off after 15 minutes and add all the oils mentioned in the list. Transfer the oils in a glass bottle. Fix a lid with a dropper so that you can take out two drops each day. It will help you to fight for extra pounds gained.

9. Grapefruit essential oil Recipe for happiness

Ingredients:

- Grapefruit essential oil – 5 drops
- Water- 2 cups
- Marjoram essential oil - 3 drop
- Bergamot essential oil - 10 drops

Directions:

Get hold of a pan in which you can add up the mentioned quantity of water. But make sure that you do not make the flame too high. It will evaporate the water too quickly. Heat on low heat till you can see visible bubbles in boiling water. Now start pouring essential oils one by one, expect the Bergamot oil. Cover the pan with a lid and wait till the water is reduced to almost half of the original quantity.

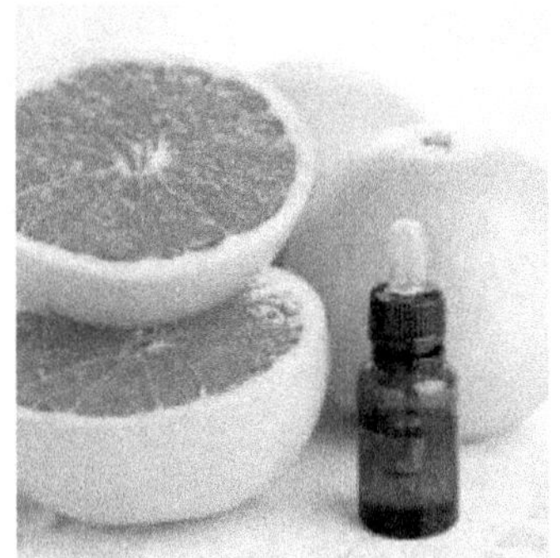

When you can reduce the quantity of water, turn the flame off and transfer the liquid to a large bowl. Let it get cooled down. When the mixture comes to room temperature, add Bergamot oil. Mix thoroughly and shift in a dark colored bottle. Place bottle in sunlight for three days. Use two drops each day, before sleeping.

10. Peace enhancing Lemon essential oil

Ingredients:

- Water- 3 cups
- Mint leaves (minced)– 5 tablespoons
- Lemon essential oil - 25 drops
- Salt– 1/2 teaspoon
- Rosemary leaves (crushed) – 1 cup

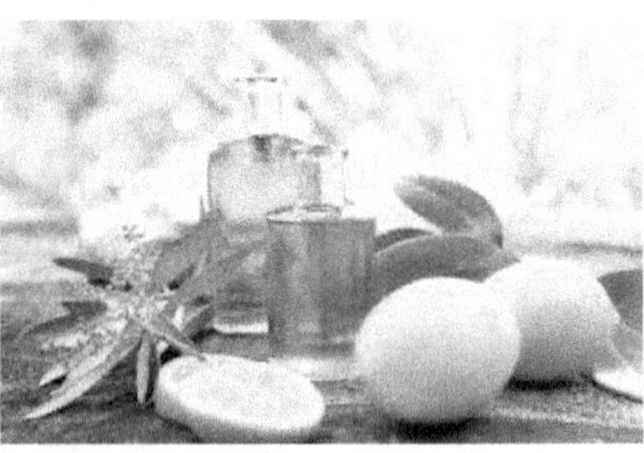

Directions:

For this recipe, first of all, get hold of a reasonable size pan in which you will be handling any of the base oil. Olive oil serves as good base oil. Put the base oil in the pan. When bubbles start to emerge out of the oil, put rosemary leaves. Cook the leaves well by stirring continuously. Wait for the cracking sound to appear. Cover with lid and switch off the heat.

Now in this mixture add mint leaves and salt. Mix excessively. Excessive heating and mixing will make a paste like material out of it. Cook well so until no coarse leaves can be seen or felt. Now take a spate glass bottle, rinsed well with warm water.

Now add the cooked mixture in that glass bottle with a layer of Lemon essential oil. Let it settle down for ten days. After that time strain out the leaves and other elements from this mixture and separate out the oil. Fill it up in a bottle and use two drops before every meal.

Chapter 2 – Get the hidden energy from essential oils

The human body is full of energy and strength but sometimes because of a hectic lifestyle and unnecessary stress over the nerves, the human body and mind gets unlimited fatigue. Essential oils can help you with hidden energy elements in every drop of essential oils.

11. Essential oil recipe for chakra balancing

Ingredients:

- ➢ Carrier Oil – 2 oz

- ➢ Rosemary Essential Oil – 10 drops

- ➢ Black Pepper oil– 4 drops

- ➢ Jojoba oil – 15 drops

- ➢ Helichrysum - 10 drops

Directions:

Mix all the oils in a bottle and stir well. Place the bottle in dark light. This perfect mixture will induce various chakras present in your body to get balanced and secured. Particularly 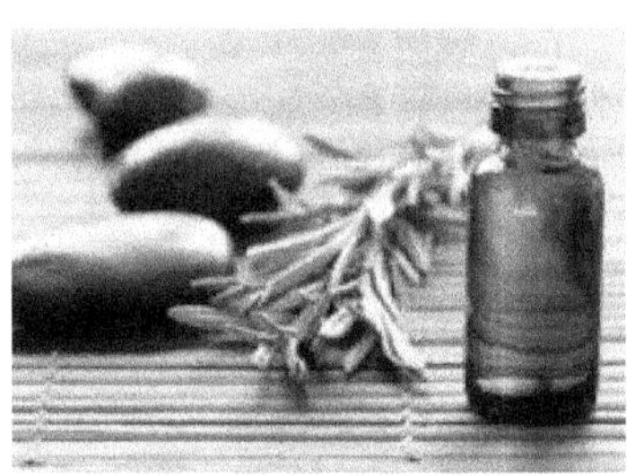 this blend of the essential oils will affect the solar chakra and you will feel energetic and full of strength.

12. Essential oil recipe for menstrual cramps

Ingredients:

- ➢ Jojoba oil - 1 ounce

- ➢ Peppermint Essential Oil - 5 drops

- ➢ Cypress Essential Oil - 4 drops

- ➢ Lavender Essential Oil - 3 drops

Directions:

Mix the oils well and add to a clean airtight bottle or container which is dark in color. Clean up the bottle with warm water. Now add all the oils and mix thoroughly. In the case of menstrual cramps apply a little over 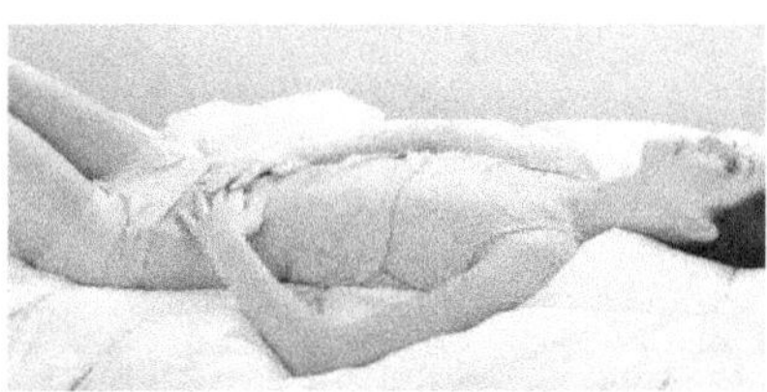 your belly and massage in circular motions. It will give a quick relief from cramps and you will feel much relaxed. You can also apply it to the tail bone for a massage or under the feet so that the pain of menstrual cycle can be reduced.

13. Essential oil recipe for gaining energy

Ingredients:

- ➢ Basil Oil – 2 oz

- ➢ Roman Chamomile – 10 drops

- ➢ Black Pepper oil– 4 drops

- ➢ Cypress oil – 15 drops

- ➢ Grapefruit oil- 10 drops

- ➢ Peppermint oil- 10 drops

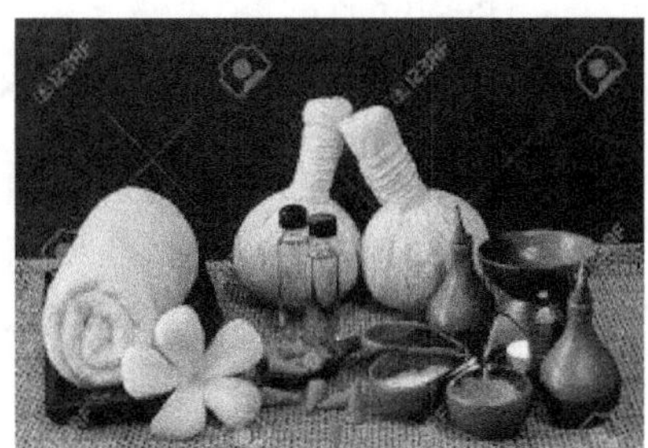

Directions:

Mix the oils well and add to a clean airtight bottle or container which is dark in color. Clean up the bottle with warm water. Now add all the oils and mix thoroughly. You can use this mixture as an inhaler. Whenever you have to spend a long hectic day or you have to carry out some challenging task you can inhaler this mixture by filling an inhaler. It can also be used by putting it over a cotton swab and inhaling the vapors.

14. Essential oil recipe for reducing depression

Ingredients:

- ➤ Bergamot oil- 1 drop

- ➤ Ylang Ylang oil- 5 drops

- ➤ Grapefruit oil- 10 drops

- ➤ Geranium oil- 20 drops

- ➤ Frankincense oil- 5 drops

- ➤ Orange essential oil- 5 drops

- ➤ Sandalwood oil- 10 drops

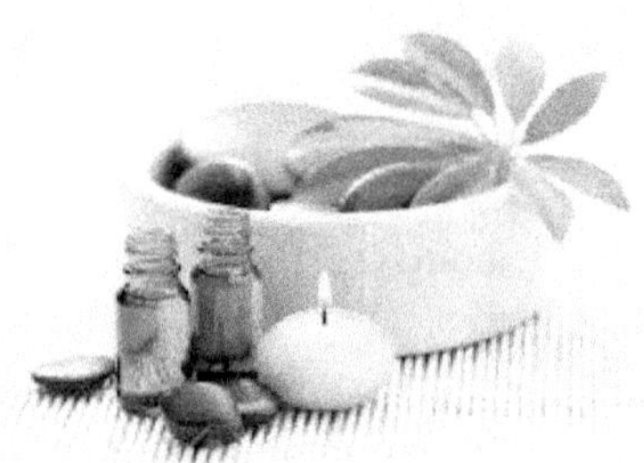

Directions:

Mix the oils well and add to a clean airtight bottle or container which is dark in color. Clean up the bottle with warm water. Now add all the oils and mix thoroughly. Fill the mixture in an inhaler and use the fumes for boosting your energy or reducing the depression levels. You can also pour it over your pillow while you are sleeping so that the fumes get induced all around the head and you get a peaceful sleep.

Chapter 3 – Get the eventual benefits hidden in every drop of essential oils

If we talk about various benefits of essential oils, it will cover major categories of beauty enhancing benefits, physical fitness, emotional wellbeing and many other household uses recipes.

Below you will find some most useful and easy to follow recipes. These recipes pertain to the most effective ones which cover a broader range of utilities for making the life easier.

15. Essential oil recipe for joint pain

Ingredients:

- ➢ Carrier Oil – 2 oz
- ➢ Roman Chamomile – 10 drops
- ➢ Black Pepper – 4 drops
- ➢ Roman Chamomile – 15 drops
- ➢ Helichrysum - 10 drops

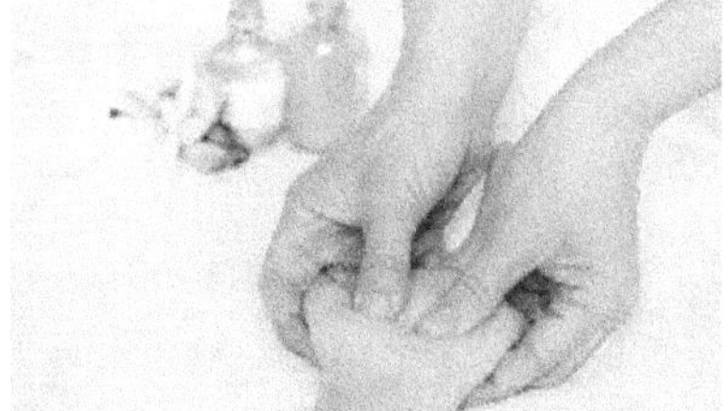

Directions:

Combine all oils together thoroughly well and keep in a container made of glass. Make sure that container is airtight and dark-colored. Now pour few drops on your palm and massage over arthritic joints or any of the joint in pain. The proper massage movements and techniques can provide a better result if you consult from your doctor. Although all the ingredients used in the mixture are best for joint pain yet in the case of any discomfort avoid using it for too long and consult your physician.

16. Essential oil recipe for scrapes and cuts

Ingredients:

- ➢ Calendula oil – 10 drops
- ➢ Grated beeswax – 1 oz
- ➢ Jojoba- 2 oz
- ➢ Lavender oil- 30 drops
- ➢ Sweet almond oil – 10 drops
- ➢ Tea tree oil - 30 drops
- ➢ Vegetable carrier - 3 Ounces
- ➢ Wide-mouth jar- 5 ounce

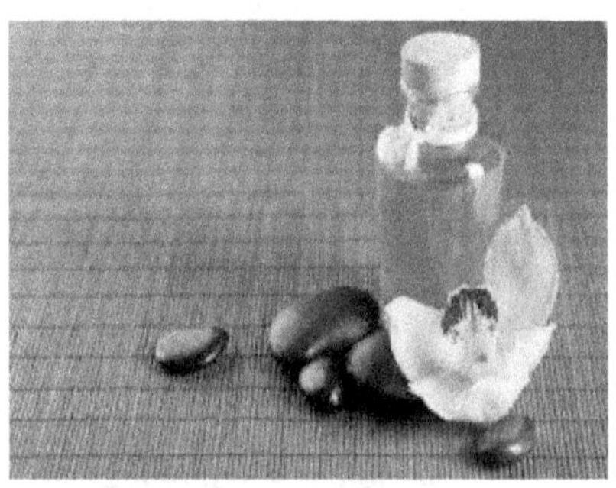

Directions:

Combine all oils together thoroughly well and keep in a container made of glass. Make sure that container is airtight and dark-colored. Now in the case of minor cuts in kitchen chores or other household chores apply this mixture. Pour just one drop and wrap with the bandage.

17. Essential oil recipe for Congestion

Ingredients:

- ➢ Eucalyptus Essential Oil- 30 drops

- ➢ Ravensara Essential Oil- 26 drops

- ➢ Peppermint Essential Oil - 4 drops

- ➢ Cotton Ball- as per needed

Directions:

Combine all oils together thoroughly well and keep in a container made of glass. Make sure that container is airtight and dark-colored. Now pour this mixture over a cotton swab. Soak the cotton swab fully and use it as an inhaler. Infusing these fumes into your nasal opening will allow you to breathe more fully and congestion problems can be cured easily.

18. Essential oil recipe for Bruises

Ingredients:

- ➢ Jojoba – 1 oz

- ➢ Sweet Almond Oil – 2 drops

- ➢ Helichrysum Essential Oil - 8 drops

Directions:

Mix the Helichrysum oil into any of the carrier oil. Now store this mixture in a dark colored or amber colored bottle. Apply on all kinds of bruises usually encountered during household chores. Rub with gentle hands.

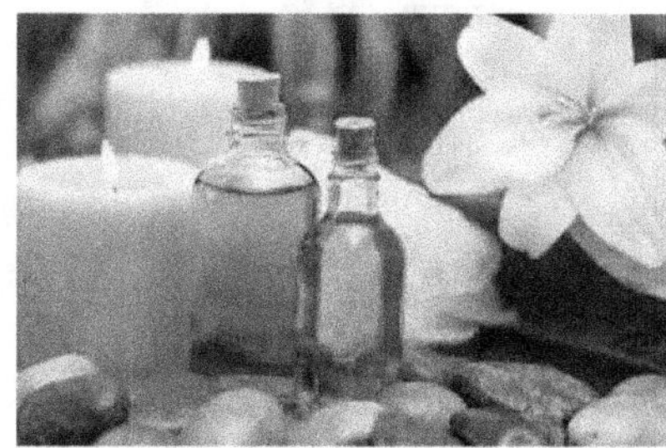

Chapter 4 – Essential oil aromatherapy- beneficial beyond your imagination

Aromatherapy is one of the latest technologies which make use of aroma of these essential oils for various benefits, including physical as well as psychological wellbeing.

19. Aromatherapy for reducing stress

Ingredients:

- ➢ Ylang Ylang Oil- 1 drop

- ➢ Jasmine Oil- 1 drop

- ➢ Grapefruit Oil - 3 drops

- ➢ Geranium Oil - 1 drop

- ➢ Frankincense Oil- 1 drop

- ➢ Bergamot Oil- 2 drops

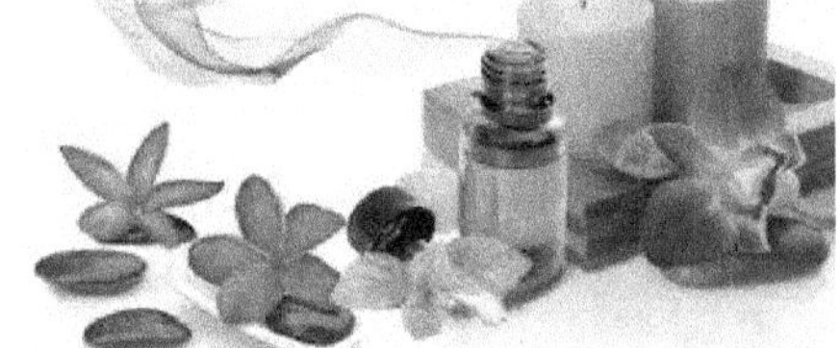

Directions:

Take a glass bottle in dark brown color. The dark colored bottle will make these oils more effective. Now add all the oils in that dark colored bottle and thoroughly mix by spinning in your hands. Now use a diffuser to add all the oils in the blender and leave in sunlight. Apply few drops over your forehead and massage well. After few days, you will feel a clear change in the intensity of stress. People who are into stress intense jobs like banking and service industry should use this oil mixture for better mental progress.

20. Aromatherapy for Emotional wellbeing

Ingredients:

- ➢ Sweet almond oil- 1 oz

- ➢ Roman chamomile - 7 drops

- ➢ Lavender oil- 5 drops

Directions:

Mix the oils well and add to a clean airtight bottle or container which is dark in color. Clean up the bottle with warm water. Now add all the oils and mix thoroughly. Roman Chamomile has a sturdy calming effect. You can use it as a massaging agent. Pour few drops of palm and massage the feet. A foot massage will add delightful and soothing effect to your 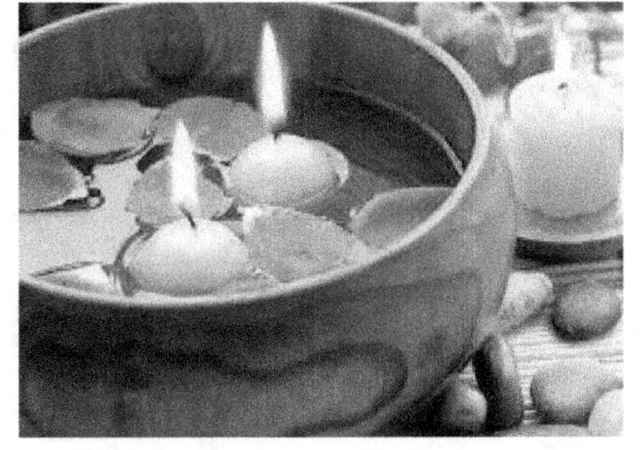 nerves. Do not go for a drive after using this massage mixture. This recipe can also be made with the help of diffuser blend. Your emotional well-being will be greatly enhanced.

21. Aromatherapy for fighting insomnia

Ingredients:

- ➢ Roman Chamomile- 10 drops
- ➢ Clary Sage - 5 drops
- ➢ Bergamot - 5 drops

Directions:

Take a glass bottle in green color. Mix together all the prescribed oils thoroughly.   This mixture will serve as an agent for fighting against insomnia.   Pour two to three drops over a cotton swab or a tissue. Place this swab inside the pillow which you use at night. Lavender Oil provides excellent relaxation leading to a peaceful sleep.

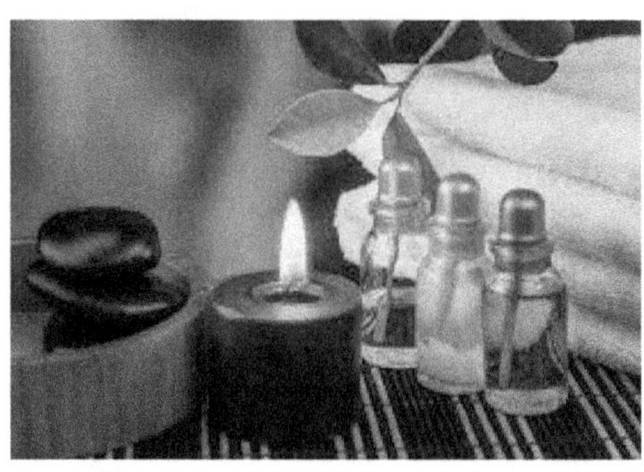

Bergamot enhances stress relief and pain. So in case your insomnia is because of some pain, this mixture will treat it as well. However using this mixture in a large amount can irritate your nerves so need to use only two to three drops.

22. Aromatherapy for Memory enhancement

Ingredients:

- Rosemary oil - 3 drops

- Lemon oil - 2 drops

- Cypress oil- 4 drops

- Peppermint oil- 1 drop

- Basil oil- 1 drop

- Hyssop oil - 2 drops

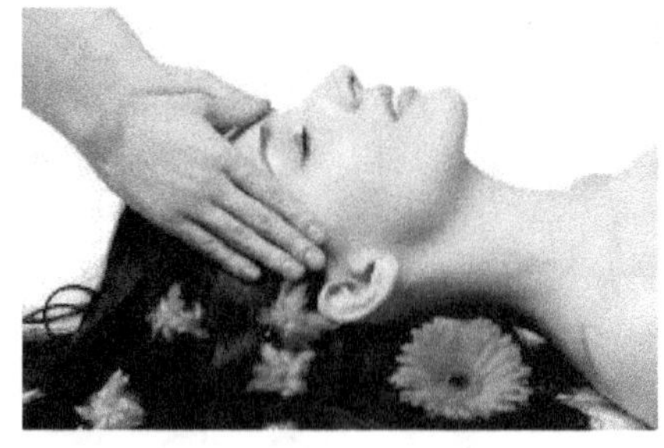

Directions:

Use a dark colored glass bottle for mixing all these ingredients in the prescribed quantity. Mix all the ingredients and leave the bottle in sunlight for ten days. Use this oil as a massager for your head and forehead. All the ingredients present in this mixture help you to enhance your memory.

These oils directly affect the brain cells which are responsible for short-term memory functions.

23. Aromatherapy for Anger reduction

Ingredients:

> - Bergamot oil- 3 drops
>
> - Ylang Ylang oil - 1 drop
>
> - Jasmine oil - 1 drop
>
> - Roman Chamomile oil - 1 drop
>
> - Bergamot oil - 2 drops
>
> - Orange oil - 2 drops
>
> - Patchouli oil - 3 drops

Directions:

Take a bottle of transparent color and 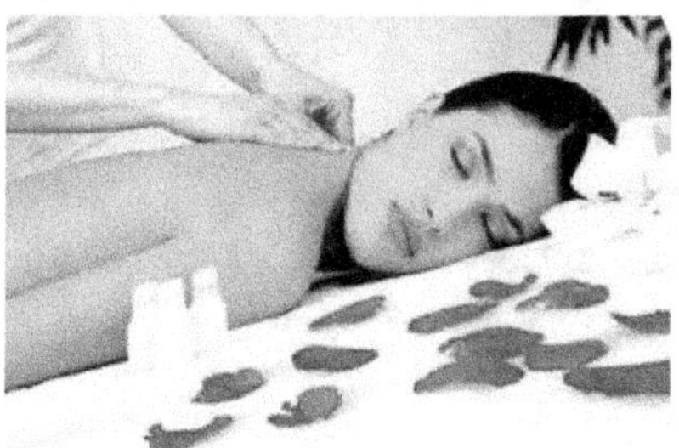 add all the ingredients in this bottle. Thoroughly mix all the ingredients and spin off the bottle well. Place the bottle at room temperature.

Placing in sunlight will allow all the extract to mix well. Now use this mixture for people who have higher levels of anger all the time. The best time for using this mixture is at night so that you can have a comfortable sleep and wake up energetic without any kind of irritation or anger.

24. Aromatherapy for Anxiety

Ingredients:

- ➢ Bergamot oil - 2 drops
- ➢ Clary Sage oil - 2 drops
- ➢ Frankincense - 1 drop
- ➢ Lavender oil - 3 drops
- ➢ Sandalwood oil - 3 drops
- ➢ Mandarin oil- 4 drops

Directions:

Take a bottle of transparent color and add all the ingredients in this bottle. Thoroughly mix all the ingredients and spin off the bottle well. Place the bottle at room temperature. Placing in sunlight will allow all the extract to mix 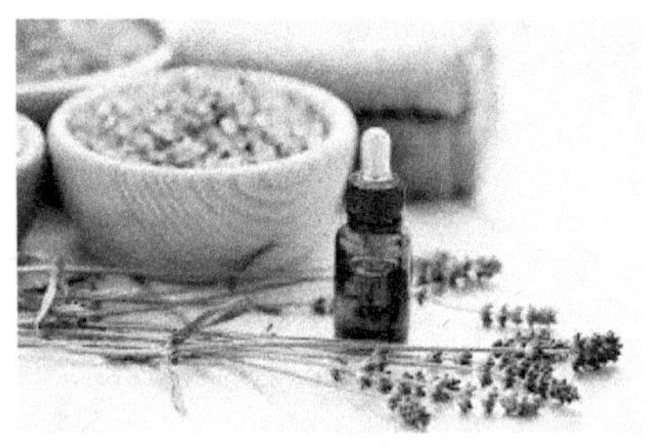 well. This mixture will serve as an anxiety relief agent. Anxiety has now become a common problem among a large number of people. So anyone of you can use this mixture as a massager at night or in the morning.

Chapter 5 – Get magnificent beauty with Essential oils

Essential oils are one of the best beautifying agents which can help you to enhance your beauty and maintain a youthful appearance. Some of the recipes are mentioned below so that you can also use these essential oils as beauty enhancers.

25. Acne care with essential oils

Ingredients:

> - Fractionated Coconut Oil – ½ oz
> - Jojoba- 1 ounce
> - Lavender Essential Oil- 6 drops
> - Tea Tree Oil - 5 drops
> - Geranium Essential Oil - 1 drop

Directions:

Take a bottle, preferably amber glass bottle. Rinse it very carefully and let it dry in open air. Now add all the essential oils one by one in the bottle and keep the lid tight. Although those bottles which have tops with rubber dropper tops cannot be utilized for storing essential oils in undiluted essential oils, but you can use it for this recipe easily.

Now spin out the bottle evenly to gently blend the oils, for two minutes. Now you can use three drops of this mixture on the face, back, neck, or any of the acne affected area. But avoid applying at eyes, nostrils, lips or inside the ears. Roll out the bottle for every use so that you can ensure effective utilization every time.

26. Facial toner Recipe

Ingredients:

- ➢ Hazel Hydrosol - 2.5 oz.
- ➢ Grapefruit Oil - 8 drops
- ➢ Tea Tree Oil - 4 drops
- ➢ Cypress Oil - 4 drops

Directions:

Put together all the ingredients in an appropriately sized bottle. Shake the bottle in circular motions so that all of the ingredients are mixed together. Make sure that you do not fill up the bottle up to the lid. It will leave some of space for shaking the ingredients before every use.

The Hazel Hydrosol present in the ingredients is an important ingredient for the toner but it can leave the toner to drying. So do not add it more than the prescribed quantity.

27. Body Lotion Recipes

Ingredients:

- ➢ Patchouli - 10 drops
- ➢ Sandalwood - 20 drops
- ➢ Carrot Seed - 5 drops
- ➢ Unscented lotion base – 8 oz

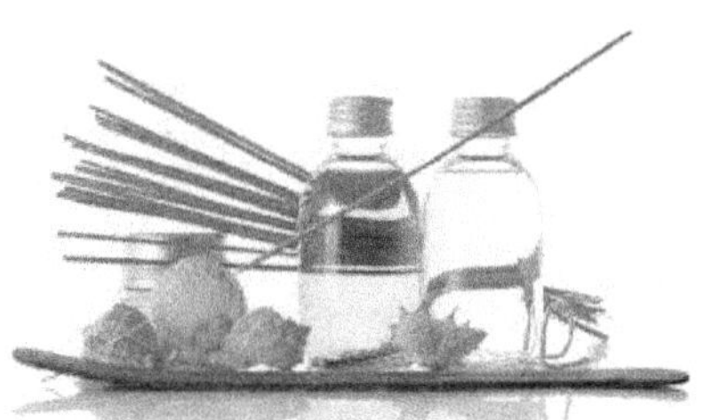

Directions:

This recipe requires the best blending of all the essential oils. For this, you can use a large bowl for thorough mixing of the ingredients. When you can see that all the ingredients are evenly mixed, you can fill up your lotion bottle with the help of a funnel.

Sandalwood present in the ingredients, adds a deep scent of the lotion whereas carrot seed oil will aid to recover the dry skin. The body lotion can be used two times a day on your face, hands, and body. It can also act as a good massaging lotion.

28. Hair conditioner recipe

Ingredients:

- ➢ Jojoba- 1 tablespoon

- ➢ Rosemary Essential Oil- 1-3 drops

Directions:

This conditioner is extremely useful as it is easiest of all to make. Take a small condiment bowl and add the Rosemary Essential Oil in it. In this recipe, you will add water in a large quantity so the rubber dropper is fine for use. Rosemary and Jojoba are efficient agents against abnormal drying of hairs.

Rosemary Oil works well against the excessive amount of dandruff. Before applying the conditioner, wet the hair with Luke warm water. Now rinse hair with conditioning blend. Leave it for twenty minutes. Rinse with water thoroughly. Make sure that the conditioner does not enter your eyes. If it enters the eyes accidently, rinse with plenty of water.

29. Body scrub recipe

Ingredients:

- ➢ Demerara Sugar – 8 oz

> Fractionated Coconut Oil- 2 tbsp

> Jojoba – 2 oz.

> Liquid Castille Soap - 1 ounce

> Rosemary oil- 1/4 tsp

> Vegetable Glycerin- 1 oz.

> Vegetable Oil- 1 Oz.

> Vitamin E Oil - 1/2 tsp

> Watermelon Seed Oil - 1/2 tsp

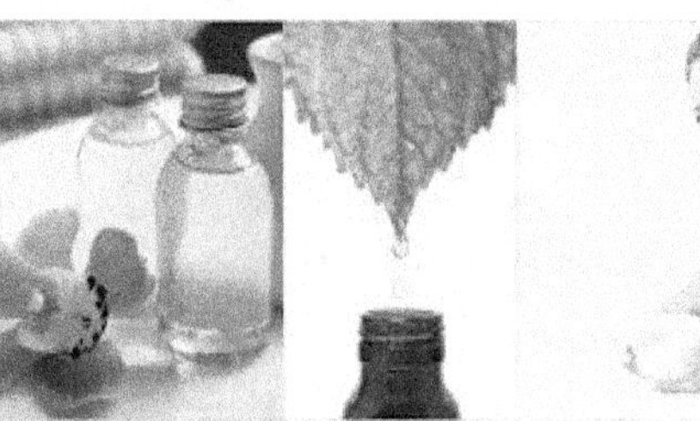

Directions:

Put sugar in a mixing bowl and grind it in an electric mixer. Do not crush sugar too fine so that it can carry on with a good scrubbing. Now in a bowl add glycerin, soils, and castile soap along with crushed sugar.

Now add essential oils and use a fork to mix well. Now use it before every bath for scrubbing your body, hands and feet. The essential oils present in the recipe will give you a glowing skin.

30. Essential oil recipe for fine cuticles

Ingredients:

> Vegetable oil – 2 oz

> Cranberry seed oil- 5 drops

> Lavender oil -5 drops

- ➢ Tea tree oil- 5 drops

- ➢ Patchouli oil - 5 drops

- ➢ Sandalwood oil- 5 drops

Directions:

For this recipe, you will need a nail polish bottle, which is not in use. Rinse through with warm water so that the entire nail posh clears away. Use a dropper to add all the essential oil one by one in the narrow-mouthed bottle.

Now make the lid tight and shake the ingredients well. Leave this mixture for fifteen days in the open air in the sunlight so that the sun rays can further enhance the effectiveness of the ingredients. Use this mixture as a remedy for healthier and fresh looking cuticles. Apply with the help of nail polish brush.

Conclusion

The best description and depiction of human life is possible through the use of natural ingredients. One of the biggest mistakes which the modern lifestyle has encountered is the unnecessary use of artificial materials and processed elements. It is because of this reason that today we have to bump into a number of different ailments and problems.

But as the experts are now exploring new ways of easing human life, they have come across in the investigation of various useful materials and botanical elements.

Essential oils are one of those miracles of creativity and utility which have hidden potentials and a number of remedial uses. Essential oils come from a variety of botanical sources and plant species, which make them utilizable in a variety of herbal and therapeutic recipes.

Just as the experts are unveiling the utilities of these essential oils many new areas are being introduced where the essential oils can prove beneficial. We all should work on this dimension to know about natural ingredients and fresh elements which can make our life much easier and healthy

. This book has touched upon only a few of these areas which can be served with essential oils. Although there can be many other uses but we have outlined only a few, which are encountered at a greater frequency. The recipes provided are also very easy and quick to follow.

The purpose for considering the simplest of all recipes is to make it utilizable for a larger number of people, who can follow these recipes in their kitchens without any special arrangements and efforts.

FREE Bonus Reminder

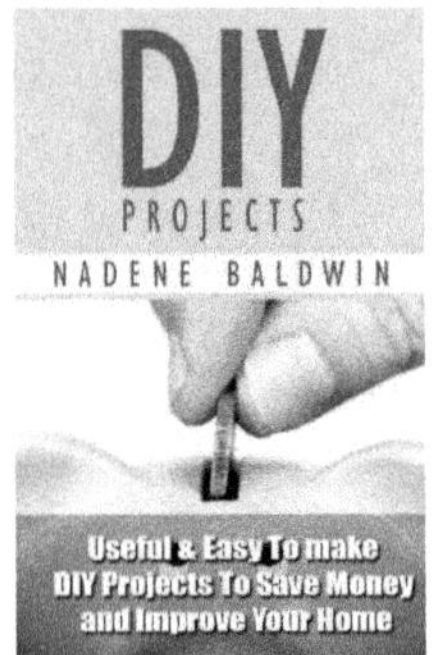

If you have not grabbed it yet, please go ahead and download your special bonus report *"DIY Projects. 13 Useful & Easy To Make DIY Projects To Save Money & Improve Your Home!"*

Simply Click the Button Below

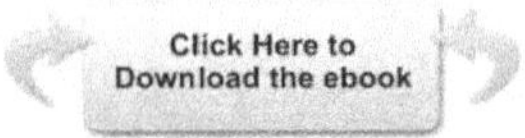

OR **Go to This Page**

http://diyhomecraft.com/free

BONUS #2: More Free & Discounted Books

Do you want to receive more Free & Discounted Books?

We have a mailing list where we send out our new Books when they go free or with a discount on Kindle. Click on the link below to sign up for Free & Discount Book Promotions.

=> Sign Up for Free & Discount Book Promotions <=

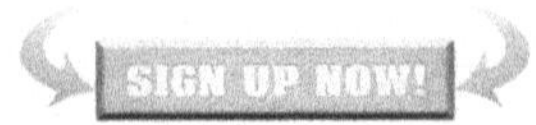

OR Go to this URL

http://zbit.ly/1WBb1Ek